Daily Yoga Routine Beginner's Guide For Happiness The Mindful & Healthy Lifestyle With Zen & Spiritual Eternity

Juliana Baltimoore

Published by InfinitYou, 2017.

While every precaution has been taken in the preparation of this book, the publisher assumes no responsibility for errors or omissions, or for damages resulting from the use of the information contained herein.

DAILY YOGA ROUTINE BEGINNER'S GUIDE FOR HAPPINESS THE MINDFUL & HEALTHY LIFESTYLE WITH ZEN & SPIRITUAL ETERNITY

First edition. June 30, 2017.

Copyright © 2017 Juliana Baltimoore.

Written by Juliana Baltimoore.

PUBLISHERS NOTES

Disclaimer

This publication is intended to provide helpful and informative material. It is not intended to diagnose, treat, cure, or prevent any health problem or condition, nor is intended to replace the advice of a physician. No action should be taken solely on the contents of this book. Always consult your physician or qualified health-care professional on any matters regarding your health and before adopting any suggestions in this book or drawing inferences from it.

The author and publisher specifically disclaim all responsibility for any liability, loss or risk, personal or otherwise, which is incurred as a consequence, directly or indirectly, from the use or application of any contents of this book.

Any and all product names referenced within this book are the trademarks of their respective owners. None of these owners have sponsored, authorized, endorsed, or approved this book.

Always read all information provided by the manufacturers' product labels before using their products. The author and publisher are not responsible for claims made by manufacturers.

Copyright 2017 InfinitYou

ALL RIGHTS RESERVED

One or more global copyright treaties protect the information in this book. This book is not intended to provide exact details or advice. This book is for informational purposes only. Author reserves the right to make any changes necessary to maintain the integrity of the information held within. This book is not presented as legal or accounting advice. All rights reserved, including the right of reproduction in whole or in part in any form. No parts of this book may be reproduced in any form without written permission of the copyright owner.

Introduction

Welcome my name is Juliana Baldec and I have been inspired by my sister Alecandra Baldec to get started with this wonderful discipline of Yoga.

I have been applying my daily yoga ritual for about three months now, but I still consider myself a Yoga beginner. I am so happy that I followed my big sister's suggestions to get started with this daily yoga ritual because it truly transformed my lifestyle, health and happiness.

I enjoy doing it so much that I decided to motivate and encourage other yoga beginners to get started with their own daily yoga ritual and routine, too.

Practising yoga does not take much time out of your schedule, and if you'd like to learn some cool time management tricks that apply to a healthy lifestyle that includes disciplines like yoga and/or meditation then I highly recommend my sister's book series that you can find on the marketplace as well.

She also was the one who inspired me to write this yoga position book for beginners because beginners are always asking her for the best poses that a beginner should get started with. She writes books that are targeted to more advanced yoga and meditation techniques so this is how I got involved in this exciting picture book project.

There are other books that talk about yoga poses, but the focus of this book is different because it does not talk about a specific yoga pose in a boring and long winded way. Who needs the whole story and history of a yoga pose anyway?

A beginner of yoga only needs a short and inspirational how to instruction so that he or she is enabled to apply the beneficial yoga pose ASAP.

This book is designed for busy yoga beginners who like to get started with some yoga poses that are specifically beneficial for beginners. The book gives a beginner the 11 essential yoga poses that are best to get started with. It also talks about the benefits of each yoga pose so that a beginner learns from the start why a specific yoga pose is good for their health and mental condition. These benefits are the true reasons a newbie needs to know about because this is the stuff that makes a newbie stick to the matter.

Each yoga pose includes some inspirational stories that I personally associate with each yoga pose, the instruction itself (think of it like a quick and to the point recipe preparation), and the specific health benefits.

I only include my favorite yoga poses that I am enjoying on a daily basis as a beginner myself and that I am having the best successes with and that I am personally feeling connected to. These are the specific poses that are giving me a healthy body and a happy mental and emotional state.

I hope you enjoy the book and I hope that you will get lots of inspiration and stimulation out of the book in order to be able to take advantage of the unlimited benefits that you can achieve with these yoga positions that you are going to discover as you go through the book.

There are seven yoga poses for beginners that are the most important to learn: the Downward Dog, Child's Pose, Bridge, Cobra, Triangle, Mountain, and Warrior Pose. Each of these poses are the building blocks for future yoga sessions and are essential to beginners. Some of these poses seemed to easy to me, but, after my first few yoga sessions, the results speak for themselves

Each and every yoga pose has its own benefits.

Enjoy your journey through the wonderful world of yoga positions!

My Favorite Yoga Quote

"Inhale, and God approaches you. Hold the inhalation, and God remains with you. Exhale, and you approach God. Hold the exhalation, and surrender to God." ~ Krishnamacharya

The Butterfly Pose

Yoga is all about uniting the mind and the body. Yoga allows us to strengthen our awareness and quiet our minds.

Being new to yoga, I like to start with the Butterfly Pose.

This pose is especially useful for starting my hectic day.

This is how the Butterfly Pose is done correctly:

Sit on your yoga mat with your back straight and your shoulders away from your ears.

Next bring the soles of your feet together, and allow your knees to fall to the floor.

Hold your feet or ankles and close your eyes.

Try to flatten your knees down toward the floor to increase your hip's flexibility.

Focus on your breath and stay in this position until you feel yourself relaxed.

I have found that allowing my mind to quiet in this position will improve my focus for the remaining positions. When I first started, my knees would stay up off the ground, but with more practice, I have been able to increase my flexibility and open my hips.

The most important benefits that come with this position are:

Health Benefits of the Butterfly Pose:

In the traditional texts it is written that "Baddha Konasana" helps destroy diseases and gets rid of extreme fatigue

The butterfly pose is stimulating the prostate gland and ovaries, the abdominal organs, the kidneys and the bladder

It also improves general circulation and stimulates the heart

The butterfly pose stretches the groins, the inner thighs and knees

It helps relieve anxiety, mild depression and fatigue

The butterfly pose soothes sciatica and menstrual discomfort

It helps relieve the sometimes very painful symptoms of menopause

The butterfly pose is a therapeutic position for flat feet, infertility, high blood pressure and asthma

Its consistent practice until late into the pregnancy is known to help ease of childbirth

Beginner's Tips of the Butterfly Pose:

Sometimes a beginner has difficulty to lower his or her knees toward the floor. If the yoga practitioner's knees are very high and if the practitioner's back is rounded, the yoga practitioner must make sure to sit on a high support (as high as a foot off the floor in some cases!)

Variations of the Butterfly Pose:

Learn to exhale and lean your torso in a forward position and between your knees. Remember to come forward from your hip joints, not your waist. Bend the elbows and push the elbows against your inner thighs or your calves. If the head does not rest comfortably on the floor, try to support your head on the front edge of a chair.

Yoga Pose 2: Cat/Cow Stretches

My favorite pose is the Cat/Cow stretch pose. I work at a computer all day long, and after eight hours at my desk, my lower back and hips can be very tight. The cat/cow stretches is a position that I can count on when I need some help to soothe my lower back pain that comes from my tough work on the computer all day long. It also helps lengthen my spine.

To do the cat/cow stretch properly, start on your hands and knees, with your knees shoulder width apart and your hands directly under your shoulders. On the inhale, round your back so your spine curves upwards.

Try to push your belly button away from the floor. On the exhale, lower your back, and raise your head. Arch your back and drop your belly to the floor. This pose helps open your spine and chest.

I have found that if I pay close attention to my breath as I am moving through this specific pose that I do get the most benefits from these stretches and this position. Allow yourself to enjoy the Cat/Cow pose and the feeling of your body opening and relaxing from a long day.

Health Benefits of the Cat/Cow Pose:
The Cat/Cow pose is stretching your neck and front torso
It provides a very gentle and soothing massage to your belly, spine and organs
Beginner's Tips of the Cat/Cow Pose:
While you are doing the Cat/Cow pose exercise do protect your neck by broadening across your shoulder blades. Make sure to draw your shoulders down and away from the ears.

Ask a friend to lay a hand just between and above your shoulder blades to assist and help you activate this area. Do this if you find it difficult rounding the very top of your upper back.

Yoga Pose 3: Downward Facing Dog

The Downward Dog pose is great for beginners because it gets the adrenaline pumping and requires every muscle in my body to participate.

To do the Downward Dog position, you start on your hands and knees and gently lift the body up in the air until the arms and legs create an upside down -V-shape.

Make sure to put your palms flat on your yoga mat and spread out your fingers. I found that spreading my fingers will help support the pose best and optimize my balance.

Hold the pose for a few easy breaths, in and out, from the nose and then release.

I also found that this pose that I enjoy very much and I think is very beneficial to beginners is helping me relax on a very deep level.

I like this pose because it is challenging but has real benefits. The downwared dog pose involves the whole body, and I often have to remind myself to breathe when I am finding myself in this enjoyable and relaxing pose.

Let's recap the pose. To start, get into a table top position on your hands and knees. Your hands should be directly under your shoulders and your toes tucked.

Bring your hips staight up, making a tall "V" shape with your body. Move your gaze toward your feet, relaxing your neck. The trick to this pose is letting your legs relax down to your heels to support your body.

As a beginner, I often find that this pose can put a lot of pressure on my wrists. If you find this to be the case, try to push back into your heels and shift your weight through your hips. Once you are able to relax when doing this pose, you'll know you are not a Yoga beginner anymore.

I am not quite there yet myself!

Health Benefits of the Downward Facing Dog Position:

The Downward Facing Dog position is Improving your posture

It strengthens your spine, wrists and arms

The Downward Facing Dog position is stretching your chest and lungs. It is also stretching your shoulders and your abdomen

It helps firm your buttocks

The Downward Facing Dog position is stimulating your abdominal organs

It also helps relieve some mild depressions, sciatica and fatigue

The Downward Facing Dog pose is a therapeutic way to combat asthma

Beginner's Tips of the Downward Facing Dog Postion Position:

If you are performing the Downward Facing Dog position, there is a tendency in this pose to "hang" on your shoulders. This results in lifting them up toward your ears and this in turn "turtles" your neck.

What you should do instead is go ahead and actively draw your shoulders away from your ears by lengthening down along your back armpits. Make sure to pull your shoulder blades toward your tailbone. At the same time make sure to be puffing your side ribs in a forward direction. If you need assistance to learn this, here is a good tip. Go ahead and lift each hand on a block.

Yoga Pose 4: Child's Pose

The next pose that I found to be very beneficial as a yoga beginner is the Child's pose. This pose is great for stretching out the back. To begin the Child's pose, lower your body onto the mat with your bottom resting on your heals. Bring your arms up and lean forward until your head is touching your knees and your arms are stretched out in front of the knees.

In my opinion this is one of the most important yoga poses you can learn because it keeps the back and torso nice and stretched out. Tight muscles make yoga way too difficult.

The Child's pose is a great transition pose for a lot of yoga positions that start from table top (on all fours). I find that this pose can serve as a resting position if I need to recenter and focus on my breath.

You should always start in table top with your hands directly under your shoulders and your knees shoulder width apart. Drop your hips down on your heels and stretch your torso down and straight. Do not move your hands as you move into the Child's Pose.

This will allow the stretch to reach all the way to your wrists as your arms elongate.

I have found that as a beginner, I am not able to fully relax into this position. If you find the same to be true, try widening your knees to allow more room for your abdomen. Allow yourself to relax in this position and concentrate on your breath.

Health Benefits of the Child's Position:
The Child's position gently stretches your back spine and your inner groins
It helps calms your brain and it also helps relieve fatigue and stress
Beginner's Tips of the Child's Position:
If you can not easily hold the feet with the hands then try the following. Go ahead and hold each foot with a yoga strap. Make sure it is looped around the middle arch.

Yoga Pose 5: Forward Fall

Another great transition pose is the Forward Fall. I use this position a lot as a resting pose between standing positions. This pose is especially useful in lengthening the spine. I particularly like this pose as it is good for loosening the neck muscles after a long day.

Stand with your feet slightly apart and your hands by your side. As you exhale, bend forward from the hips and let your torso gently fall forward. Allow your knees to bend so that you can fully lengthen your spine. Try to rest your torso on your thighs and bring your hands to the floor. Go only as far as is comfortable.

As a beginner, I often have to modify this pose. I use a block to rest my hands on, as I am unable to comfortably rest my hands on the floor. You can also adjust the bend in your knees to your comfort level. This pose is wonderful for stretching the hamstrings and calves and relieving tension in the lower back.

Health Benefits of the Forward Fall Position:

The Forward Fall position is calming your brain and it helps relieve mild depressions and stress in a wonderful way

It is stimulating your kidneys and liver

The Forward Fall position helps stretch your hamstrings, your hips and your calves

It also helps strengthening your knees and thighs

The Forward Fall position helps improve your digestion

It helps relieve any symptoms of menopause

The Forward Fall position helps reduce anxiety and fatigue

It helps relieves insomnia and headaches

The Forward Fall position is a very therapeutic means to help combat asthma, infertility, high blood pressure, sinusitis and osteoporosis

Beginner's Tips of the Forward Fall Postion Position:

To help increase the stretch in your backs of the legs, do bend the knees slightly. Imagine that the sacrum is sinking deeper into your back of your pelvis and make sure to bring your tailbone closer to your pubis.

Then against this resistance, push your top thighs back and your heels down and straighten your knees again.

Be careful not to straighten your knees by locking them back (you can try pressing the hands against your back of each of your knees to provide some resistance).

Yoga Pose 6: Warrrior One

Warrior one is all about control. I try to do the pose in stages to increase my balance while getting the most out of the stretch. This pose is great for strengthening the knees and elongating the body.

Step your feet out side with your toes pointing forward. Place your hands on your hips and turn your right foot out 90 degrees. Let your right knee follow as you turn your torso to the right. Take a moment to find your balance and on the next exhale, bend your right knee until your knee is directly over your ankle.

Don't bend too far. You should be able to barely see your toes beyond your knee. To add another element to the pose, raise your hands over your head, with your palms together, and bring your gaze to your hands. Maintain this pose for several breaths and then repeat on the other side.

You should feel the stretch through your left leg and up through your wrists. It took me a while to work up to raising my arms in this pose. Keeping your hands on your hips and your gaze straight ahead will still allow you to stretch your lower body. Keep at it until you can relax into the pose.

Health Benefits of the Warriror One Position:

The Warrior position stretches the lungs, chest, shoulders and your neck, groins (psoas) and belly

It strengthens your arms and shoulders as well as the muscles of the back

The Warrior One position stretches and strengthens your ankles, calves and thighs

Beginner's Tips of the Warrior One Position:

Remember the following. When your front knee is bending into this pose, a yoga beginner has the tendency to tip his or her pelvis forward, which

duck-tails the coccyx and which compresses his or her lower back.

Keep in mind that as you perform step 2 of theWarrior One pose, be sure to lift your pubis toward your navel and also lengthen your tail toward the floor. Make sure to take notice of the following. As you are bending your knee, continue to lift and descend your two bones, keeping the top rim of your pelvis parallel to the floor that you are standing on.

Yoga Pose 7: Pigeon Pose

The Pigeon pose is one of my favorite stretches. It opens the hips and thighs and is great for relieving tension that can build up from sitting all day. I know that after a long day, this pose really feels good!

From table top, move into the Downward Facing Dog position. From here, raise your right leg until it is in a straight line with your body. In one fluid motion, bring your right leg up and under your body, bending the knee and lowering the hips. Your right knee should be near your right hand, with your knee pointing out to the side.

Both hips should be touching the floor. You can bring your gaze up to open the lower back, or bend your elbows until you are resting on your forearms and bring your forehead toward the floor. This will deepen the stretch in your hips. To return to the Downward Facing Dog position, curl your toes on your left foot and press your hands into your yoga mat. Lift your hips and then move your right leg back even with your left one. Repeat the pose on your left side.

As a beginner I find that I cannot quite get both hips square to the floor. If this is the case, place a block underneath the right thigh to help support your body. If your hips aren't square, you'll put too much strain on your lower back.

I am still working at fully opening my hips so that the block isn't necessary.

Health Benefits of the Pigeon Position:
The Pigeon position helps opens your hips and also the fronts of the upper thighs.

Beginner's Tips of the Pigeon Position:
Walk your hands back so your body is vertical over your hips. Don't forget to breathe and to press into your hands to take some weight out of the hips and roll your hips square to the front of the yoga mat. Take your time to do this and keep the front of your body very long and very open.

Yoga Pose 8: The Tree Pose

The Tree pose is a balance pose that helps strengthen your concentration. In the beginning, I struggled with this pose, but now I am able to hold the position for longer.

Stand with your feet close together and your hands on your hips. If you have trouble balancing, do this pose close to the wall to protect you from falling.

When you are ready, lift your right leg off the floor and bend at the knee. Grasp your right ankle and place the bottom of your foot against your left inner thigh. Your right toes should point toward the floor. If necessary, you can modify the pose by placing the sole of your right foot against your left calf muscle. Do not let your right foot rest against your knee. Find your balance, and when you are steady, bring your palms together in front of your heart. If you are able, raise your hands above your head. Keep your gaze forward. Maintain this pose for several breaths. Then repeat on the left side.

The Tree pose is a peaceful pose and is very useful, not only in improving balance, but also quieting your mind and centering your awareness. I still keep my hands in front of my heart, rather than raising them up, as I find my balance is better in this pose. But I will keep practicing until I am able to fully execute the pose. I hope you will keep practicing as well!

Health Benefits of the Tree Position:

The Tree position strengthens your thighs, your calves, your ankles and your spine

It stretches your innter thighs and your groins and your chest and shoulders

The tree position improves your sense of balance

It also relieves sciatica and it reduces flat feet

Beginner's Tips of the Tree Position:

If the raised foot tends to slide down your inner standing thigh as you perform this position, put a folded sticky yoga mat between your raised foot sole and your standing inner thigh.

Yoga Pose 9: The Bridge Pose

The Bridge pose is another essential yoga pose for beginners. It literally is a bridge into learning various other yoga positions later in yoga sessions. The Bridge pose is very easy to do. All you have to do is lay down on your back and put your arms to the side.

Bend the knees and slowly roll the torso up. The most important thing to remember about this and any yoga position is to hold your core muscles as tight as possible. This will optimize the effectiveness of the yoga pose.

Health Benefits of the Bridge Position:
Physical Benefits of the Bridge Position:

The Bridge position helps stretch your neck, chest, shoulder, spine and hip flexors

It also stimulates your lungs, your thyroid gland and your abdominal organs

The Bridge position improves your digestion and your circulation

It is known to build endurance

Therapeutic Benefits of the Bridge Position:

The Bridge position calms the whole body in general

It alleviates the built up stress and mild depressions

The Bridge position reduces your headache, your back pain, your fatigue, your insomnia and your anxiety

It helps relieves symptoms of asthma as well as hypertension/high blood pressure. It also helps relieve symptoms of menopause, sinusitis and osteoporosis

Energetic Benefits of the Bridge Position:

Energetically speaking, the Bridge position helps activate everyone of your chakras. It helps get your body's energy moving and especially the first chakra, the third chakra, the fourth chakra, and your fifth chakra.

Yoga Pose 10: The Cobra Pose

The most challenging pose for beginners to learn is the Cobra pose. This is because of the amount of muscle strength it takes to execute this pose properly.

First, you lay on the mat on your stomach and your nose to the floor. Put your palms of your hands on your yoga mat, and using the core muscles, lift the front part of the body until the arms are extended. This is a tough pose because every time I do it I want to use my arms to lift myself up. The arms are more for balance and support. The core should be doing most of the work.

Health Benefits of the Cobra Position:

The Cobra position helps strengthens your spine

It helps stretch your chest area and your lungs. The Cobra pose also helps your abdomen and your shoulders, too

The Cobra pose helps firm your buttocks

It helps stimulate your abdominal organs and it even is good for relieving your stress levels

The Cobra position does help relieve your stress levels and your fatigue levels

It also opens your heart and your lungs and soothes the whole body

The Cobra position helps sooth sciatica and it is a very effective and therapeutic way to heal asthma

Traditional texts are claiming that this Bhujangasana position does increase your body heat. The position is also known to be able to destroy diseases and to awaken kundalini.

Beginner's Tips of the Cobra Position:

As a beginner to yoga you should never overdo the backbend of this position. To find out about the height at which you can comfortably work out and avoid straining the back, make sure to take the hands off the floor for a short moment. If you do it like this the height you find will be through your body extensions.

Yoga Pose 11: The Triangle Pose

The most challenging pose for beginners to learn is the Cobra pose. This is because of the amount of muscle strength it takes to execute this pose properly. First, you lay on the mat on your stomach and your nose to the floor. Put your palms of your hands on the mat, and using the core muscles, lift the front part of the body until the arms are extended. This is a tough pose because every time I do it I want to use my arms to lift myself up. The arms are more for balance and support. The core should be doing most of the work.

Health Benefits of the Triangle Position:

The Triangle pose helps stretch your legs, your muscles around the knee, your ankle joints, your hips, your groin muscles, your hamstrings, your calves, your chest and your shoulders and spine

It strengthens your knees and legs, your ankles, your obliques, your abdominals and back

The Triangle position helps stimulate your function of abdominal organs and it also relieves your stress levels

It improves your constipation and your digestion

The Triangle pose does help to alleviate the symptoms of menopause and back pain

It is also used in a therapeutical manner to combat anxiety, neck pain, infertility and sciatica

How To Follow Up With The Poses

During every session of yoga, I would start with the Mountain pose. You stand with your feet hip width apart and your arms to your side. The point is to stand tall, chest erected, to represent a mountain.

Coming out of the Mountain pose, you can go right into the Warrior pose. To do the Warrior pose, simply just stretch one leg out from the Warrior Pose stance and bend the knee until it is just over the heal. Bring the arms to the side and keep the arms parallel to the knee and body.

Every yoga pose of beginners has it benefits. The seven that I just talked about are the ones that beginners will need to know in order to further their yoga training.

At first, I was skeptic at whether or not yoga would be an effective work out, but, after the first session I was exhausted and felt great. Yoga releases all toxins out of the body and leaves you feeling rejuvenated and refreshed.

Health Benefits of the Triangle Position:

The Mountain pose helps improves your posture, but it also helps strengthen your thighs. It is known for its powerful healing results and it can help relieve your back pain

Beginner's Tips of the Mountain Position:

Practice the moutain position with your back pressed against the wall so that you can truly feel the alignment that is happening

If you need, you can also use a block between your thighs. Squeeze the block with your thighs and roll the block slightly backward in order to feel the engagement and the rotation of your thighs.

Body Mind Connection

If you practice yoga, it is important to know how meditation and yoga connect and what it provides to the body. Being in a state of meditation is being in a high state of yoga. The connection is part of achieving a healthy lifestyle and spiritual fulfillment. Basically meditation helps you get the most out of yoga but it is so much more than that.

The two states of spirituality are closely linked. Meditating can help you do yoga better and doing yoga gives you a better capacity to meditate. The focus of meditation skills is on clearing the mind. The focus of yoga skills is on the physical well-being. Connected together the benefits are endless. There are both physical and mental benefits to yoga training when combined with meditation practices.

Meditation not only relates to yoga but is actually an integral part of yoga training. Meditation is connected with the various yoga postures. The postures help you concentrate so you can better benefit from both practices. It is part of the mental aspects of yoga that enable you to concentrate intently on what your body is doing. This brings about calmness of mind. It takes amazing concentration levels to be able to do some of the more advanced poses in yoga.

Dhyana or meditation is one of the limbs of yoga. Some of the other significant limbs are Pranayama which is the focus on breathing, Pratyahara which is the withdrawal of senses and Dharana which is concentration. These closely related limbs work together to bring a state of harmony to your being through the connection of yoga and meditation.

Dhyana involves the process of emptying your mind. You silently focus on various chakras or energy points in the body to achieve a sense of meditation and calm. Meditation techniques allow a user to let go. You are able to disengage your body from your thoughts in order to truly relax and discover serenity.

Pranayama is concentrating on each breath and guiding it to where it needs to be in order to achieve the most benefits. You are in essence breathing your life source. Each breath should be evenly drawn where you take in as much breath as you let out. Balanced breathing puts you in a meditative state. Pranayama is arguably one of the most important aspects of yoga training. It definitely helps you transport to the place you need to be when doing yoga.

Pratyahara is turning your senses inward and letting go of the outside senses. It is a connection between the inner and outer forces of the spirit. The control of senses makes us achieve a greater sense of awareness of ourselves and the spirituality around us.

Dharana basically means focusing on one thing. It keeps the mind in a state of attentiveness without any outside influences. It is needed for yoga to be able to hold the poses. Many of the yoga poses are held for a long period of time. It may look simple but it requires a mental state that is achieved by meditating.

The various limbs of yoga work together and one leads into the other while also seeming to be interconnected. The goal is achieving a balance of mind, body and spirit which can better be accomplished when yoga and meditation are combined. The two very much work hand in hand.

The connection of yoga and meditation techniques offers many health benefits. Yoga for health is not a modern trend as some believe; the numerous benefits have been keenly aware of for over 5,000 years. It keeps you in tune with your mind and body in a variety of ways.

Yoga and meditation provide a unique balance which allows you to stay healthy and mentally fit. Your body becomes stronger and more flexible. The various poses are toning and strengthening while at the same time relaxing. This dual benefit helps maintain both a healthy mind and healthy body.

Yoga lowers blood pressure and improves circulation. Deep breathing enhances proper blood supply. The improved blood flow cleanses the body and provides the much needed flow of oxygen. Muscles and other body parts need oxygen to function properly and yoga gives the muscles just that.

Because both yoga and meditation focuses on breathing, lung function noticeably improves. Respiratory problems are relieved because of the controlled breathing exercises. Yoga classes often prescribed to heart patients as a form of healing.

Yoga cleanses and heals the body moving you to a higher state of well-being. Over time, practicing yoga and meditation teaches the mind to become serene. People who practice yoga and meditation are more centered and grounded and in control of their bodies becoming more aware of their inner spiritual self.

You will find that energy levels are increased. In fact there are specific poses geared to increase energy and reduce feeling of tiredness and fatigue. Additionally, the deep breathing exercises encourage oxygenation of dormant energy cells that may exist in the body.

Yoga is very therapeutic. It helps in managing chronic pain issues and actually reduces pain levels. Your muscles loosen up and your body is more supple and flexible. The more use muscles get, the less painful it will be to use them. Yoga skills also coax the body to release natural pain killers.

You will find that by practicing yoga along with meditation techniques will reduce anxiety and feelings of depression. Participating in yoga skills actually result in the body secreting hormones that help the body cope with depression. Yoga is considered to be a natural mood enhancer so it will relieve feelings of depression. It is also beneficial in relieving anxiety and the combination of deep breathing exercises along with muscle strengthening postures and the inner focus of meditation work wonders in improving how you feel.

Yoga and meditation work together to give you a sense of inner peace. A more calm and stress free existence will result from experiencing how meditation and yoga connect and work together. You will walk away feeling refreshed and renewed from practicing the various skills and techniques involved in yoga.

Make sure to take at least 5 minutes out of your day and integrate some blissful meditation minutes into your daily lifestyle because not only will this benefit your Yoga routine in the long run, but a daily meditation practice will benefit your inner and outer self with in so many different ways.

Once you find your own way of zen which should be everyone's goal of the life journey, you will truly understand what is meant by this body mind connection because like everything in life you have to experience it for yourself in order to be able to attach meaning to it.

If you have not yet started your meditation journey, make sure to check out the second book that is included in this compilation because the meditation poems from A to Z called "Zen Is Like You" do help you with the discovery of meditation. They show you many ways of Zen so that you can go ahead and reflect upon them and get in touch with your own blissful way of Zen.

Conclusion

My goal with this picture yoga poses book for beginners was to give the novice just enough information to enable them to make an informed decision as to whether or not they will opt to include these easy to practise yoga beginner positions into their daily lifestyle and benefit from such a daily yoga ritual in terms of health, peace of mind, happiness and unlimited possibilities!

I hope I have delivered and fulfilled this goal.

I also hope that this yoga position picture book is going to stimulate you mentally and that it is going to motivate and encourages you to make yoga part of your future lifestyle.

I encourage you to take note of the many benefits that come with each yoga position and to take the book with you as you go and apply each new yoga position that is covered in the book.

Just keep the book on your mobile device next to your yoga mat and go through one yoga position at a time and as you progress. The book is intended to be used as a mental stimulation and to motivate you to take action at the same time.

I tried to make it as effortless, entertaining, inspirational and easy to use and consume as possible.

I hope you will use and consume the content whenever you need some ready to go yoga pose instructions. If you really use it as it is intended to be used (use it as you go through the positions and keep it close during your yoga exercise time!) it is a very powerful way of discovering the unlimited world of yoga!

Remember, all you have to do is open the book and start with the first yoga position. Go through all of them and apply them on a daily basis as you see fit and depending on the health benefits that you are looking to achieve.

You just need a bit of time (even 5 minutes per day is enough!) to be able to apply at least one yoga position to your lifestyle. You can increase the time as you go and you can repeat one or more positions (depending on your own situation) during the day.

Remember, you can achieve the maximum of health benefits from yoga just by using these simple to apply yoga positions for beginners that you find included in this book and without spending a fortune on yoga instructions.

Once you have achieved your own yoga goal by following these easy to follow basic yoga positions for beginners, you can go ahead and learn the more advanced yoga positions and bring your body and mind in unison.

If you have enjoyed this book and would like to learn more advanced yoga and meditation lessons, you can check out some of Alecandra Baldec's yoga and meditation lifestyle books below.

Alecandra is my sister and she has inspired me to get started with yoga myself and to discover the wonderful world of yoga!

She has also encouraged me to create this book and do it in a way that makes it valuable for a yoga beginner in terms of the specific benefits (so that you do understand why yoga is so beneficial for you!) that come with each yoga position and in terms of making the discipline of yoga effortless and

5 minute quick in terms of instructions and usability (you can use the book next to your yoga mat and just use it like you would use a cookbook). Using the book pretty much like a cookbook makes your daily yoga exercise a 5 minute quick and enjoyable process.

Using modern, mobile, interactive and time saving technology is really how you are enabled to make this yoga ritual work for you. Use this book like you would use a cookbook (this "cookbook" technique really makes this beneficial yoga lifestyle possible for you!).

Alecandra taught me all of these cool 5 minute time management and usability techniques that she likes to include in her own meditation and yoga ritual to make it work for her. Integrating these tips into your own yoga ritual is exactly how you enable and empower yourself to transform your life into a lifestyle with yoga!

You can learn more about Alecandra's cool ways of integrating yoga and meditation into the daily lifestyle without any effort and in 5 minutes! She really knows how to integrate these beneficial disciplines into one's daily lifestyle.

If you like to learn more about integrating yoga and meditation in an effortless way into your own daily lifestyle even if you only have 5 minutes to do so, please check out her book series by typing in Alecandra Baldec into your favorite search engine, goodreads, or online marketplace.

Helpful Yoga Resources

https://www.udemy.com/yoga-with-perumal-course-series-1[1]

http://www.yogajournal.com
http://www.abc-of-yoga.com
http://yoga.about.com
http://www.myyogaonline.com
http://www.yogawiz.com
http://www.yoga.com
http://www.corepoweryoga.com
http://www.yogacards.com
http://www.thesecretsofyoga.com
http://www.kripalu.org
http://www.bikramyoga.com
http://www.himalayaninstitute.org/yoga-international-magazine
http://www.yogadownload.com
http://yogatothepeople.com
http://www.yogatoday.com
http://www.yogashakti.org/surya-namaskar

---

1. https://www.udemy.com/yoga-with-perumal-course-series-1

http://www.yogatreesf.com
http://www.ashtangayoga.info[2]
http://www.sivananda.org
http://www.bandhayoga.com/flyarounds.html
http://www.anusara.com
http://www.iyiny.org
http://www.yogalearningcenter.com/welcome/index
http://www.poweryoga.com
http://fingeryoga.com
http://www.artofliving.org/us-en
http://www.kundaliniyoga.org
http://www.mkprojects.com/pf_Tibetan-Rites.htm
http://www.yogaglo.com
http://www.laughteryoga.org

---

2. http://www.yogatreesf.com

Did you love *Daily Yoga Routine Beginner's Guide For Happiness The Mindful & Healthy Lifestyle With Zen & Spiritual Eternity*? Then you should read *Daily Meditation Beginner's Guide From Happines & Good Life to Stress Release, Relaxation, Healing, Weight Loss & Zen* by Juliana Baltimoore!

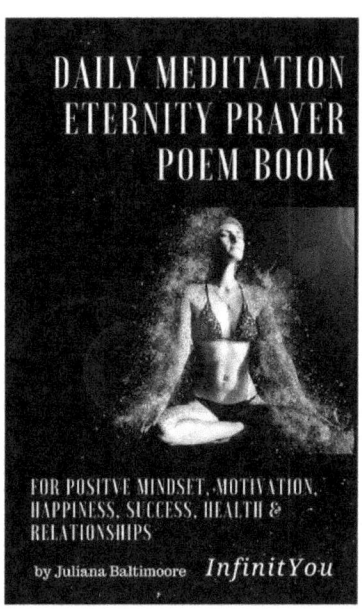

InfinitYou's Daily Meditation Beginner's Guide From Happines & Good Life toStress Release, Relaxation, Healing, Weight Loss & Zen combines soul & spirit searching, flexibility & the modern lifestyle, and powerful meditation techniques in a very strategical and unique way and creates the ultimate effortless system for everybody who wants to enjoy a life with meditation. This book has been created for beginners and advanced users alike and it is perfect for people who have tried to integrate meditation into their life but have failed because of time constraints and modern life complexities. The book reveals the latest insights into the mind-body consciousness connection and how to make meditation work in todays world where time has become such a valuable resource. Especially watch out for the secret success ingredient that is going to be the connecting part and the reason why her system works so well for people who always lack time. This secret technique makes this system work for everyone who would love to enjoy a lifestyle with meditation. Many people who would love to lead a lifestyle with meditation are unable to go through with it because they don't have enough time and therefore think meditation is not for them and then they give up. This system closes the gap and resolves this problem forever and helps you to achieve a proper daily meditation ritual that is real. Heck, you can do this. The key here is to give this system a chance and learn how to benefit from this secret success ingredient. Why? Because it is easy to do and it is effortless to do and best of all it only takes 5 minutes to do. Everyone who really wants to achieve a true meditation lifestyle is able to apply this and there are no excuses why you can't do it. It takes no effort and time at all! Heck you can even do this if you have no time for meditation during the day and if you crawl into bed at 2 pm in the morning after a long day of work. No matter what your working hours look like or how constrained your time schedule looks like, Alecandra is going to show you the way out of it and even if it is 2 pm in the morning and you have not had time to do your meditation up to now. This system is for everyone who is looking for a lifestyle with meditation. No matter how much time you got on hand, you can still follow this system and be successful with meditation. Once you follow this extremely easy and effortless system that is for the most extreme cases only going to take 5 minutes per day, you will be able to achieve a proper daily meditation ritual. Being able to apply this daily meditation ritual equals living a lifestyle with meditation which is going to bring you to the ultimate goal itself: unlimited possibilities, happiness, and unlimited health and mental benefits, and so much more... If you would like to enjoy a truly effortlessly system that makes a true meditation lifestyle really possible for you, try this one secret ingredient technique and you will never want to go to the backwards way of doing meditation the old fashioned way. You can follow this meditation system if it is 2 pm in the morning and you have not been able to do your meditation work before bedtime. You might be a busy person and have many time constraints and in this case this system will work wonders for you. If you truly want a life that includes meditation but have not found the right combination that works for you on a daily basis, you must absolutely know about Alecandra's secret ingredient that will give you the 5 minute key to a true meditation lifestyle - a meditation lifestyle that is so valuable and enjoyable to live! Start living a lifestyle with meditation today and if you apply this system your life will benefit from unlimited possibilities on every level of life. See you on the other side where you can transform your lifestyle into a truly stimulating and exciting daily meditation ritual!

Also by Juliana Baltimoore

Meditation Book For Beginners: 15 Daily Strength Training & Home Workout Yoga Routines For Beginning Yogi Students

Daily Meditation Beginner's Guide From Happines & Good Life to Stress Release, Relaxation, Healing, Weight Loss & Zen

Daily Yoga Routine Beginner's Guide For Happiness The Mindful & Healthy Lifestyle With Zen & Spiritual Eternity

Daily Meditation Eternity Prayer Poem Book For Positve Mindset, Motivation, Happiness, Success, Health & Relationships

Superfoods Recipes: Chicken Soup Recipes For Cold Recovery, Healthy Chicken Noodle Soup Recipes, Holistic Healing Chicken Recipes & Homemade Healing Noodle Soup With Chicken

31 Blender & Mixer Smoothie Recipes For Rapid Weight Loss

The Poetry Book For The Paleo Lifestyle

21 Green Fruit And Vegetable Smoothie Snacks: Green Fruit Yogurt Smoothies, Vegan Desserts & Herbal Veggie Bullet Blender Drinks

Blender Cookbook: 60 Blender Cocktails Recipes For Body Cleanse & Detox, Energy, Vitality & Rapid Weight Loss

Fasting Book For Health, Fitness, Weight Loss & Detoxing 11 Juicing For Beginners Recipes With delicious & Healthy Fruit & Vegetable Juices

Juicing Recipes Book For Vitality, Energy, Health And Fitness Nutrition 14 Healthy Clean Eating & Drinking Juice Cleanse Recipes

Smoothie Recipe Book To Gain Energy & Detox 17 Smoothie Bowl Recipes, Cleanse Drinks & Blender Mix Recipes To Feel Stronger

Fitness Cookbook: 60 Healthy Nutrition Blender Recipes, Vegan Gourmet Recipes, Juicing Drinks, Dessert Recipes & Healthy Ice Creams For Wellness, Health & Happiness

Juicing Recipe Book: 27 Epic Juice & Blender Recipes For Health, Detox, Weight Loss, Energy, Strength & Vitality

Scrumptious Paleo Desserts: Low Fat Low Cholesterol Dessert Recipes For A Healthy, Happy, Lean & Clean Eating Lifestyle

Weight Loss Juicing Recipe Book: Epic Juicer Mixer Blender Recipes For Loosing Body Fat, Body Cleansing & Detox

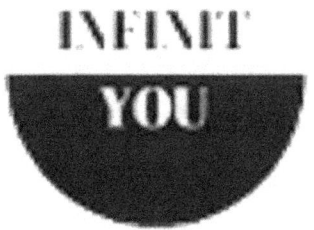

About the Publisher

InfinitYou is a hybrid general interest trade publisher. One of the first of its kind InfinitYou publishes physical books, electronic books, and audiobooks in various genres. Our publications are meant to educate, edify and entertain readers of all walks of life from babies to the elderly. Home to more than twenty imprints such as Infinit Baby, Infinit Kids, Infinit Girl, Infinit Boy, Infinit Coloring, Infinit Swear Words, Infinit Activities, Infinit Productivity, Infinit Cat, Infinit Dog, Infinit Love, Infinit Family, Infinit Survival, Infinit Health, Infinit Beauty, Infinit Spirituality, Infinit Lifestyle, Infinit Wealth, Infinit Romance, and lots more.

www.ingramcontent.com/pod-product-compliance
Lightning Source LLC
LaVergne TN
LVHW020500080526
838202LV00057B/6069